The Art of
NATURAL BEAUTY

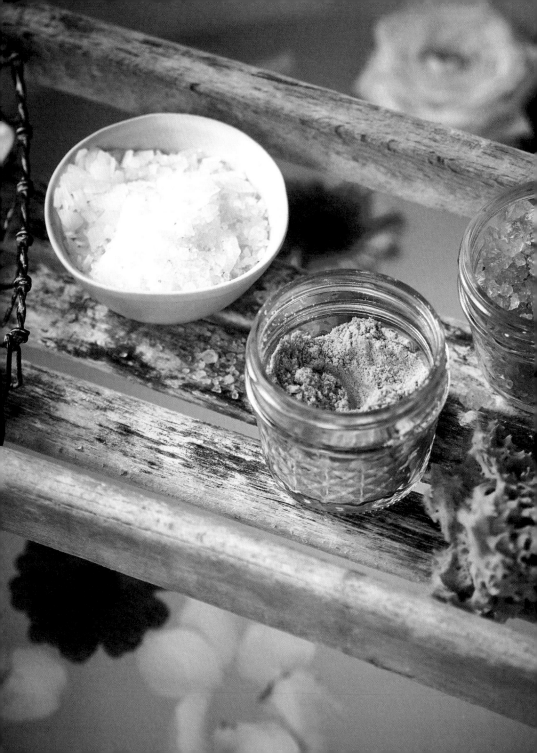

The Art of
NATURAL
BEAUTY

Homemade lotions and potions
for the face and body

Rebecca Sullivan

photography by Nassima Rothacker

Kyle Books

For my besties Fran, Emma, Anne, Kate, Biela, Beata, Niki, Carolina, Rachel, Lucy and Sibila. Natural Beauties inside and out.

First published in Great Britain in 2018
by Kyle Cathie Limited
Part of Octopus Publishing Group Limited
Carmelite House, 50 Victoria Embankment
London EC4Y 0DZ
www.kylebooks.co.uk

10 9 8 7 6 5 4 3 2 1

ISBN 978 0 85783 478 2

Project Editor: Tara O'Sullivan
Copy Editor: Anne Sheasby
Editorial Assistant: Sarah Kyle
Designer: Laura Woussen
Photographer: Nassima Rothacker
Illustrator: Chrissy Lau
Stylists: Rebecca Sullivan and Rachel de Thample
Prop Stylist: Agathe Gits
Production: Lisa Pinnell

A Cataloguing in Publication record for this title is available from the British Library.

Colour reproduction by ALTA london
Printed and bound in China by 1010 International Printing Ltd

The information and advice contained in this book are intended as a general guide to using plants and are not specific to individuals or their particular circumstances. Many plant substances, whether sold as foods or as medicines and used externally or internally, can cause an allergic reaction in some people. Neither the author nor the publishers can be held responsible for claims arising from the inappropriate use of any remedy or healing regime. Do not attempt self-diagnosis or self-treatment for serious or long-term conditions before consulting a medical professional or qualified practitioner. Do not undertake any self-treatment while taking other prescribed drugs or receiving therapy without first seeking professional guidance. Always seek medical advice if any symptoms persist.

CONTENTS

Introduction

The chemical-laden product I was smoothing all over my cheeks contained at least 13 things I couldn't pronounce nor could I have told you what they were. I felt a bit of a hypocrite after years of banging on about what we should and shouldn't put in our bodies. There I was, standing in the bathroom putting blusher on my cheeks, and I had a sudden realisation that I was saying one thing about what I ate and doing the opposite with what I put everywhere else.

On average, women use around 12 personal care products a day. If you add that up by way of individual ingredients if they're shop-bought, potentially that's well over 100 different ingredients going into your body via your skin. If even just a quarter of those are chemicals, that's a lot of rubbish going into your blood stream. Eek. And when there are no legalities in the beauty industry, like there are with food and drink, anything could be going in there. Mainly synthetic fillers, water and alcohol. I can think of better things to do with the alcohol.

If being better to your body isn't enough to get you across the line, what about our animal friends and all the testing that cosmetic companies still do? Or think about the effect on our environment, all those chemicals, and all that packaging? And if none of that works, then consider this. A blusher on the high street costs on average around 25 times more than the one in this book. See that happy dance your purse is doing. Yep, I can see it too!

I realise that organic produce and products can be more expensive but where possible try to use them – after all it's going into your skin. If you can't get organic, try to use a natural version or unsprayed produce. Make friends with your local farmers at a market or your neighbours for their flowers. You can always swap them for a jar of handmade body butter.

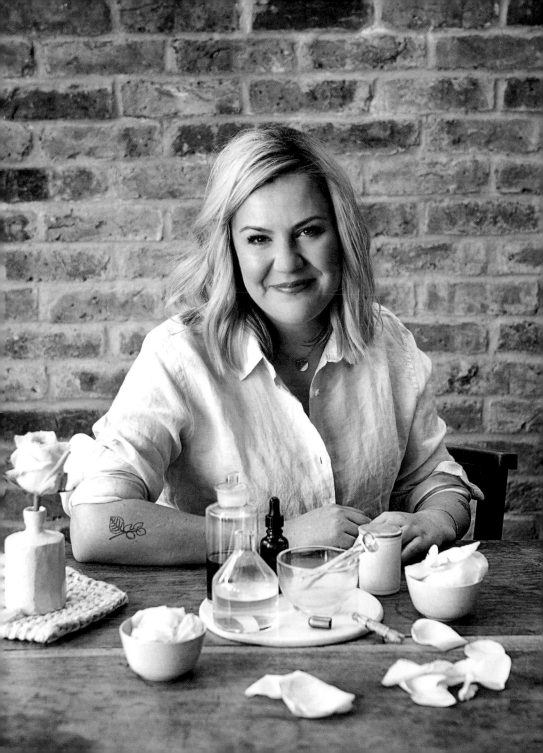

Chapter One

skincare

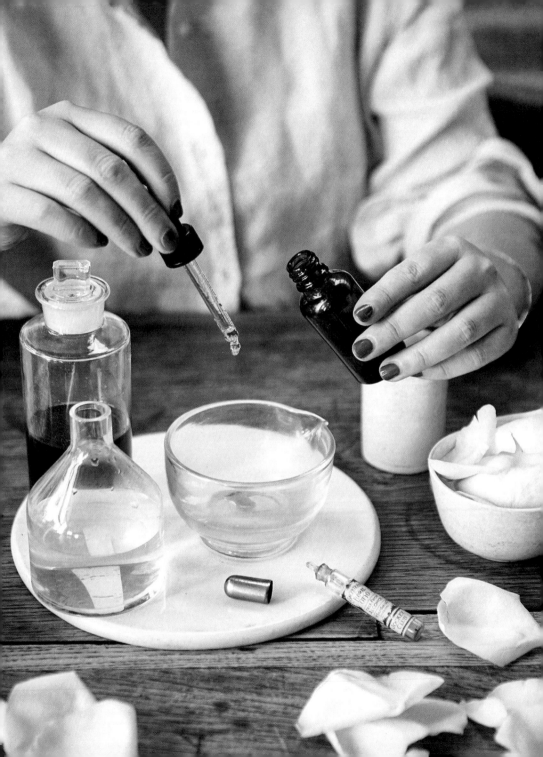

To extend the shelf life of this oil further, to about 6 months, add 2 drops of pure vitamin E oil.

Avocado & rose face oil

Perfect for dry skin. Avocado and rose are both super nourishing and hydrating, making this the perfect moisture treatment whilst you sleep. Rose is said to be anti-ageing, so here's hoping that we wake up having shed a few years as well.

MAKES 100ML

6 tablespoons avocado oil
1 teaspoon rosehip essential oil
2 teaspoons rose water
8–10 drops of rose essential oil

sterilised 100ml bottle

Place all the ingredients in a sterilised small bottle and shake to mix. Keep in a cool, dry place or in the fridge for up to 3 months (see Tip above).

To use, wash and dry your face before bed, then put a few generous drops of this oil on your fingertips and rub them together to warm the oil. Apply the warm oil to your face, leaving it to soak in while you sleep.

Milk & honey facial wash

Buttermilk is soothing, so this facial wash is great for sensitive skin. Honey is anti-fungal, anti-microbial and nourishing. The mixture of elderflowers and violets helps with soothing skin too, as they are both emollients, which means they help the skin to retain moisture.

MAKES 150ML

150ml buttermilk

1½ tablespoons raw honey

1 teaspoon dried elderflowers
  or 2 teaspoons fresh

1 teaspoon dried violets
  or 2 teaspoons fresh

sterilised 150ml jar

Place all the ingredients in a small saucepan and set aside for a few hours (off the heat) to begin macerating.

Next, bring gently to the boil over a low heat. Once the mix has reached the boil, remove from the heat and leave to cool.

Once cool, strain into a sterilised jar and close the lid. Store in the fridge for up to a week and use twice a day (morning and night) to cleanse the skin.

I've used buttermilk here as it's better for sensitive skin, but you can use full-fat milk if you prefer.

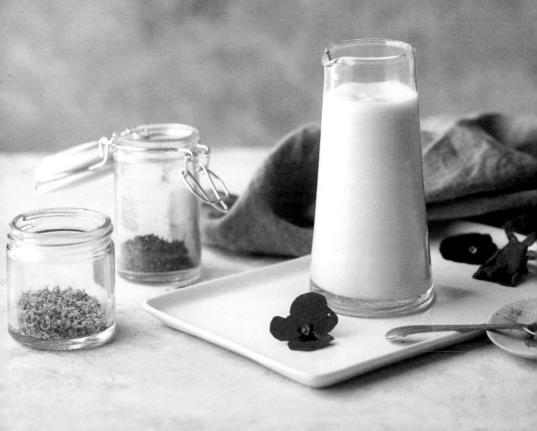

Almond & orange blossom cleanser

This cleanser smells like summer. It also tastes like summer. It is quite a thin cleanser so it's best used with a cloth, or it can be used as a toner instead of a cleanser. If all else fails, it makes a fabulous breakfast.

MAKES 250ML

125g raw unblanched whole almonds
3 tablespoons raw honey
225ml filtered water
5 tablespoons orange blossom water

muslin cloth
sterilised 250ml jar

Blitz the nuts in a high-speed blender until very finely chopped. Transfer the nuts to a bowl and gradually beat in the honey with a fork or whisk, then do the same with the filtered water and orange blossom water until combined. Cover with a cloth or tea towel and leave overnight at room temperature.

The next day, strain the mix through some muslin (squeezing as you go) into a sterilised jar and close the lid. Store in the fridge for up to a month.

Use day and night as a face cleanser by putting some on a cotton cloth or cotton pads, wetting your face and rubbing the cleanser in a circular motion. Rinse with warm water.

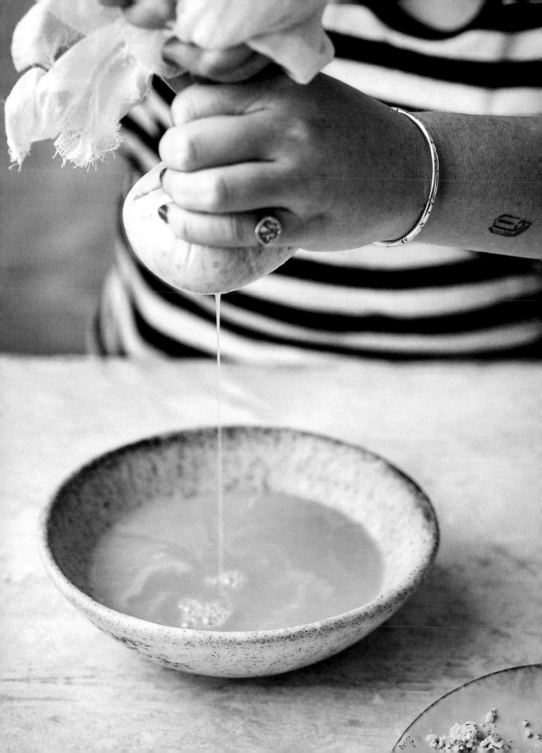

Face masks five ways

I love face masks – what a great opportunity to have a lie down and let the mask work its magic, then rinse with warm water and moisturise as normal. Because they have no preservatives in them, these may be a little runny or might not stick to the face perfectly.

Turmeric & honey

Curcumin (the main compound in turmeric) helps to soothe skin irritations, treat burns and assist in repairing sunburn. It can also help with the healing process of wounds. Honey has so many health benefits too, including being excellent for acne and inflammation. Please note that using turmeric may stain some people's skin temporarily. I recommend using this face mask before bed and using a sugar scrub afterwards.

MAKES 1 FACE MASK

1 tablespoon finely grated fresh turmeric root or ground turmeric
1 tablespoon raw honey
1 tablespoon natural yogurt

Mix all the ingredients together in a bowl, then apply to a clean, dry face. Lie down and let it dry for about 10–15 minutes. Wash it off with a cloth using warm water. Any leftover can be kept in the fridge or given to a friend – it will keep for up to 3 days.

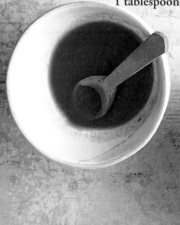
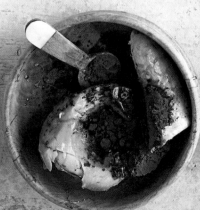
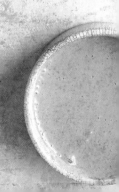

Kakadu plum

Kakadu plums have the highest natural source of vitamin C in the world and are native to Australia. I have been using this powder for everything and I truly believe it is magical. You can buy it online and it will be sent worldwide. A little tip, when you're feeling run down, mix a teaspoonful with some water and take it as a shot for a few days, letting it work its magic.

MAKES 1 FACE MASK

2 teaspoons Kakadu plum powder
a few drops of water

Mix the plum powder and water together in a tiny bowl to make a thick paste. Apply to a clean, dry face, then leave for 10–15 minutes. Wash it off with warm water.

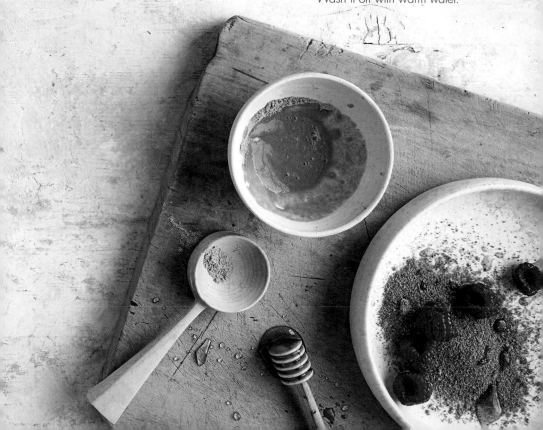

Berry good

Berries and honey sound like the beginning of a delicious smoothie. Not only good for your insides, but good for your outsides too. Berries are high in antioxidants and vitamins, and honey has more benefits than I can list, but a couple are its anti-bacterial and anti-microbial properties (oh, and it never goes off). If a little happens to fall in your mouth while you're enjoying this mask, lucky you!

MAKES 1 FACE MASK

25g fresh berries (such as blueberries, blackberries or raspberries, or a mixture)
1 teaspoon raw honey
1 teaspoon coconut sugar

Mix and smoosh all the ingredients together in a small bowl. Apply to a clean, dry face, then leave for 10–15 minutes. Wash it off with warm water.

Choc, avo and banana

Who doesn't have a few ageing bananas lying around that are destined for smoothies? Next time, try this instead. I also always eat half an avocado at a time and hate the other half going brown by the next day, so this is the perfect way to use it up.

MAKES 1 FACE MASK

½ banana, peeled
½ avocado, stoned and peeled
1 teaspoon raw honey
1 teaspoon raw cacao powder

Mix and smoosh all the ingredients together in a small bowl. Apply to a clean, dry face, then leave for 10–15 minutes. Wash it off with warm water.

Bloody mary

Eating tomatoes provides natural sun protection from UV rays, as well as promoting youthful skin. Tomatoes are rich in lycopene, which is a powerful antioxidant. So get them onto your skin too, minus the vodka.

MAKES 1 FACE MASK

1 ripe tomato
squeeze of lemon juice

Blitz the tomato in a small blender. Add the lemon juice and stir. Apply to a clean, dry face and leave for 10–15 minutes. Wash it off with warm water, then leave your face un-moisturised after applying this particular face mask, otherwise your pores will block.

Porridge face scrub

Oats are so fantastic at removing dead skin cells and they are great for sensitive skin too. They have properties that ease skin irritations, such as eczema, when eaten or put directly onto the skin.

MAKES 1 APPLICATION

1 tablespoon rolled or porridge
    oats
1 tablespoon raw sugar
1 tablespoon raw honey
½ teaspoon ground cinnamon

Mix all the ingredients together in a small bowl until just combined. Using a circular motion, massage the mix onto a clean face. Rinse with warm water, dry and moisturise as normal.

Pink & green clay cleanser

When I was a teenager, I remember my mum using the Body Shop's Japanese cleansing grains. I used to sneakily use them in the shower and loved the feeling left after a good, yet gentle, scrub. This is my take on those with the same (nostalgic) results. It's fantastic for your face and décolletage.

Pink clay is great for dry and sensitive skin types. It aids in reducing irritation and inflammation from aggravating skin conditions, such as acne. Green clay is rich in minerals and allows for far more absorption of dirt, dust, oil, contaminants and make-up than any other clay. It helps to draw out impurities from the skin and brings fresh blood to damaged skin cells, helping to tighten and revitalise pores. It is excellent for clearing problem skin, too, so the two of them combined are a great pimple bust-up!

MAKES 460G
(enough for 15–20 applications)

75g rolled or porridge oats
75g amaranth
30g raw brown rice
15g dried thyme
15g dried sage
125g green clay
125g pink clay

airtight container

In a spice blender, blitz the oats, amaranth, rice and herbs together to make a medium–fine powder (or to your preference). Add both clays and mix in. Transfer the mix to an airtight container and store in a cool, dry place for up to 3 months.

To use, put about 2 teaspoons of the clay mix into the palm of your hand, wet with a little water to make a paste, then use the paste to scrub your skin, massaging gently over the skin in a circular motion. Rinse with warm water and dry.

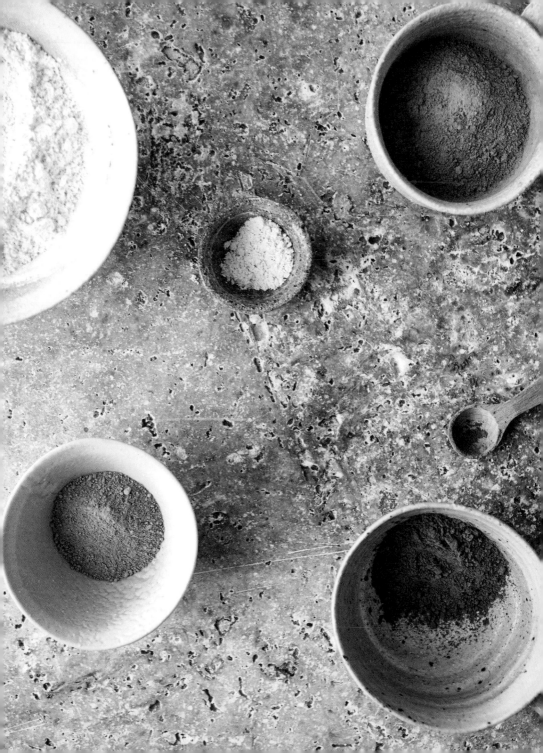

Five ways to say bye-bye puffy eyes

Puffy eyes are caused by excess fluid in the connective tissues around the eyes. These five quick, easy and natural solutions will mean you can get rid of those puffy, dark circles. Be sure to keep your eyes closed with all these eye treatments. Some will be drippy and may run into your eyes, but all of them are non-toxic and won't harm you. If your eyes do become irritated, you may be allergic or sensitive to the ingredients, so just rinse with warm water.

Chamomile tea

Chamomile is used as a natural anti-inflammatory and antioxidant, which is what makes it perfect for puffy eyes.

Make yourself a cup of chamomile tea using 2 teabags. Let the teabags cool down and then lie down and place the bags over your closed eyes for 10 minutes. You can also do this with loose leaf tea – simply brew the tea, then dip cotton pads or scraps of clean cotton cloth into the tea. Leave to cool, then place these over your eyes in the same way as the tea bags.

Potatoes

Potatoes reduce puffiness. It sounds crazy but it works. Don't ask any more questions, just try it.

Slice a potato into thin rounds, large enough to cover your eyes, then wet them. Lie down and place the slices over your closed eyes for 10 minutes.

Eyebright

Eyebright has been used medicinally for thousands of years. It has properties that brighten tired eyes and can reduce inflammation and itchiness, so is perfect for hay fever.

Pour 300ml water into a small pan, add 20g dried eyebright and bring to the boil. Simmer for 5 minutes, then remove from the heat and leave to cool. Once cool, strain into a sterilised jar. Use by soaking cotton pads (or pieces of clean cotton cloth, big enough to fit over each eye) in the eyebright liquid. Lie down and place the pads over your closed eyes for 10–15 minutes.

Ring a ring o' roses

Roses are anti-ageing and have a tightening effect. Over time they can reduce the appearance of wrinkles too. Great for reducing the crow's feet around your eyes.

In a pestle and mortar, smoosh together a handful of unsprayed fresh rose petals with a tiny drizzle of rose water. Lie down, close your eyes and pat a little scoop of the mix onto each eye. Leave for 15 minutes, then rinse off with warm water. Don't make it too watery, otherwise it won't stay on your eyes.

Egg whites (not in an omelette)

Egg whites tighten your skin and shrink pores too, so whilst you're lying down, massage a little onto your face.

Simply whisk 2–3 egg whites in a bowl until stiff peaks form. Lie down, close your eyes and pat a little scoop onto each eye. Leave for 15 minutes, then rinse off with warm water.

Honey & rose toner

Honey and roses smell utterly delightful together and they both have incredible healing and anti-ageing properties. Honey is the most gentle exfoliant and is naturally anti-bacterial, making it perfect for oily skin and blocked pores. Use this toner to remove the last residual dirt after a face wash and prior to moisturising. You can also carry it in a little spritz bottle in your handbag for a pick-me-up and hydration burst when travelling.

MAKES 150ML

140ml warm water (just warm, not boiling, otherwise you'll kill the good properties in the honey)

1–2 teaspoons raw honey

2 teaspoons rose water

10–12 drops rose essential oil

if you have oily skin, add

1 teaspoon lemon juice or apple cider vinegar

if you have dry skin, add

1 teaspoon almond or olive oil

if you have combination skin, add

1 teaspoon lemon juice or apple cider vinegar AND 1 teaspoon almond or olive oil

sterilised lidded jar or small spray bottle

Pour the warm water into a small bowl, add the honey and stir until dissolved. Add all the remaining ingredients and stir to combine. Decant into a sterilised lidded jar or small spray bottle and leave to cool. Store in a cool, dark place or in the fridge for up to 3 months.

You can swap the rose water and rose essential oil for orange blossom water and orange essential oil. Orange is said to rejuvenate skin cells.

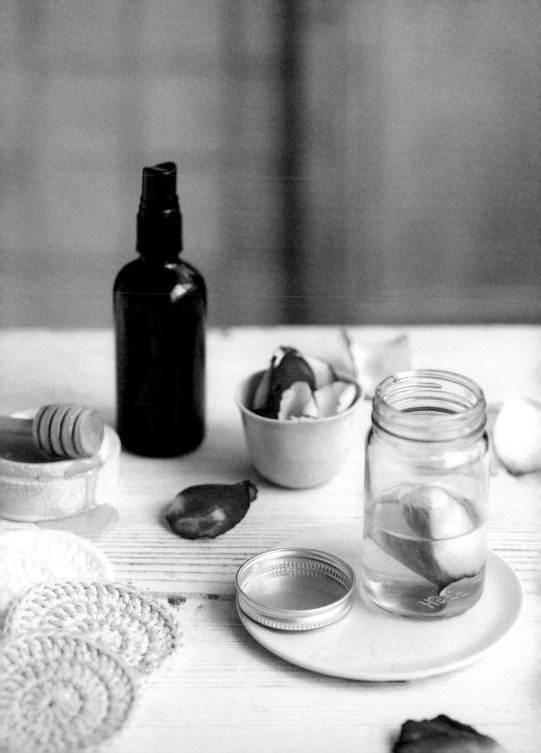

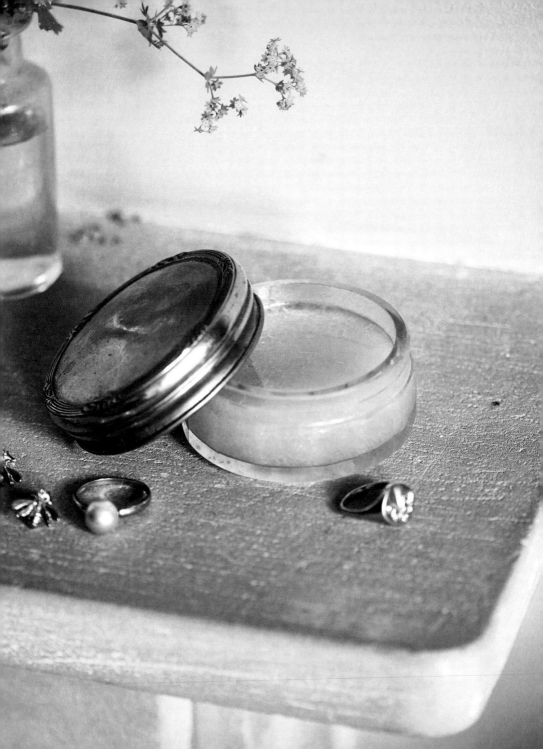

Elderflower night cream

Elderflowers are one of my favourite flowers for eating and drinking and now using on my skin. If you can't get elderflower water, you can easily make your own (see recipe below). Elderflowers are moisturising, so they are a great addition to this face cream.

For the elderflower water

MAKES 200ML

5 small handfuls fresh elderflowers or 3 small handfuls dried (if you're picking your own fresh flowers, be sure to gently shake out any little critters that might be hiding in there)
250ml boiling water

sterilised bottle or jar

If using fresh flowers, pick them when fully opened. Place the flowers in a heatproof bowl and cover with the boiling water. Cover the bowl with a tea towel and leave overnight.

The next day, strain the flavoured water into a sterilised glass bottle or jar, seal and label. Store in a cool, dark place for up to 6 months. Once opened, store in the fridge and use within a few months.

For the night cream

MAKES 170ML

6 tablespoons aloe vera gel
3 tablespoons coconut oil
1 teaspoon vitamin E oil
1 tablespoon apricot kernel or avocado oil
1 tablespoon Elderflower Water (see above)
4 drops of rose essential oil (optional)

sterilised jar

First, mix the aloe vera gel and coconut oil together in a bowl. Add all the other ingredients and mix until combined. Cool and use a hand-held blender to emulsify. Transfer to a sterilised jar and close the lid. Store in a cool, dark place for up to 3 months.

Use liberally on your skin at night before bed, gently rubbing it into the skin. It's also good to use on dry skin during the day.

Rosy face moisturiser

Roses are the greatest for skin care. They are active, hydrating and anti-ageing, so this moisturiser is perfect for dry skin. More than that, roses just smell utterly delightful. Search out the roses that actually smell – they are few and far between in the shops these days, so maybe make friends with your neighbour (the one with the scented roses) and swap them for a jar. The amount of extra oil you will get from the roses is dependent on their moisture level.

MAKES 200ML

4 large handfuls of fresh rose
    petals (any colour), unsprayed
    and perfumed
250ml avocado or extra virgin
    olive oil
10g beeswax
2 teaspoons vitamin E oil
10 drops of rose essential oil

wide-mouthed jar
sterilised jar, for storage

Start by shaking off any wee critters inside your rose petals. Put the petals into a wide-mouthed jar and cover with the avocado or olive oil. Use a wooden spoon (or smaller jar that fits inside the larger jar) to bruise the petals (drawing out some of the moisture). Put the lid on the jar. Leave in the sunlight (inside, but not somewhere too hot – just a place where it can get sunlight) for a couple of weeks. Strain the oil into a bowl and discard the petals.

Put the strained rose oil and the beeswax into a double boiler over a low heat and heat until melted and combined. If you don't have a double boiler, then instead use a heatproof bowl set over a pan of barely simmering water (making sure the bottom of the bowl doesn't touch the water underneath).

Remove from the heat and leave to cool a little, then stir in the vitamin E oil and rose essential oil. Pour into a sterilised jar and leave to cool completely before putting the lid on. The mix will emulsify like coconut oil does, but will melt when touched. Keep in a cool, dark place for up to a month.

Use as required, gently rubbing into your skin.

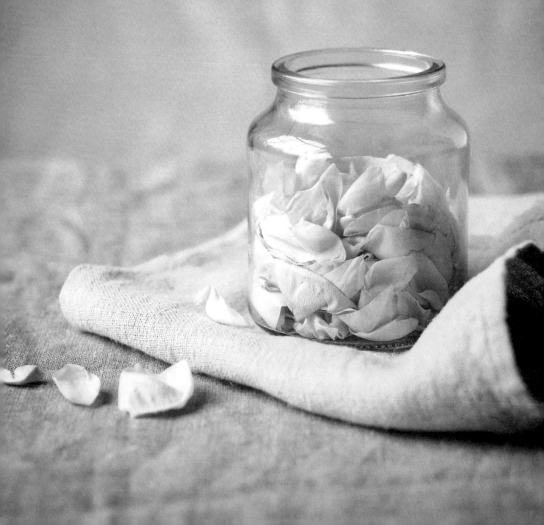

Check the jar of petals after
the first week. If you can't see
any change in the oil level, add another
50-100 ml of oil.

Chapter Two
make up

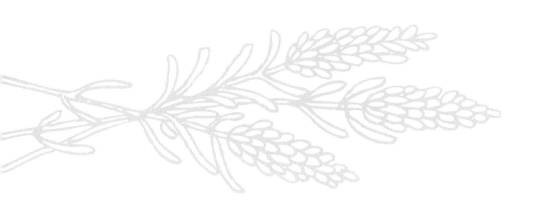

Lavender lip scrub

This is the perfect little primer for your lips once every couple of weeks, or when needed. Great for those of you who wear a bit of lippie, but for those that don't you'll still love this anyway.

MAKES 30ML

1 tablespoon coconut sugar
1½ teaspoons raw honey
1½ teaspoons avocado oil
2–4 drops of lavender essential oil

sterilised small container or jar

Mix everything together in a small bowl, then transfer to a sterilised small container or jar and cover with the lid. Store in a cool, dark place for up to 6 months.

Use by rubbing a little of the scrub on bare lips for 20 seconds or so. Rinse with warm water and then apply lip balm or your lipstick.

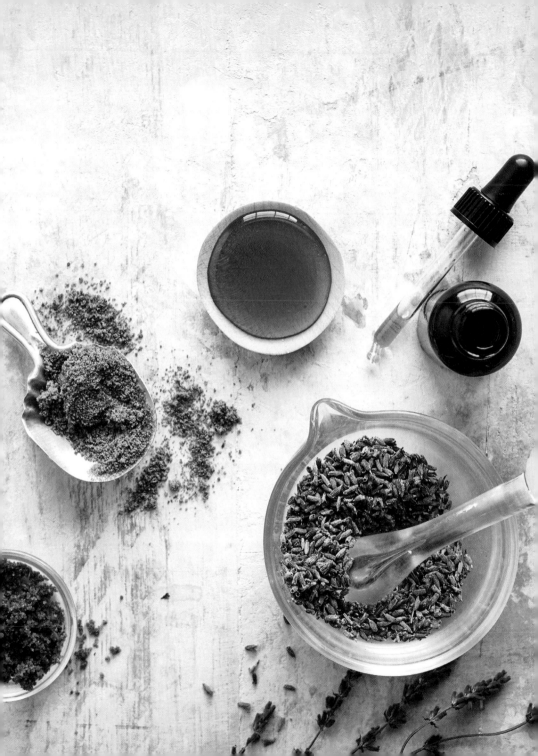

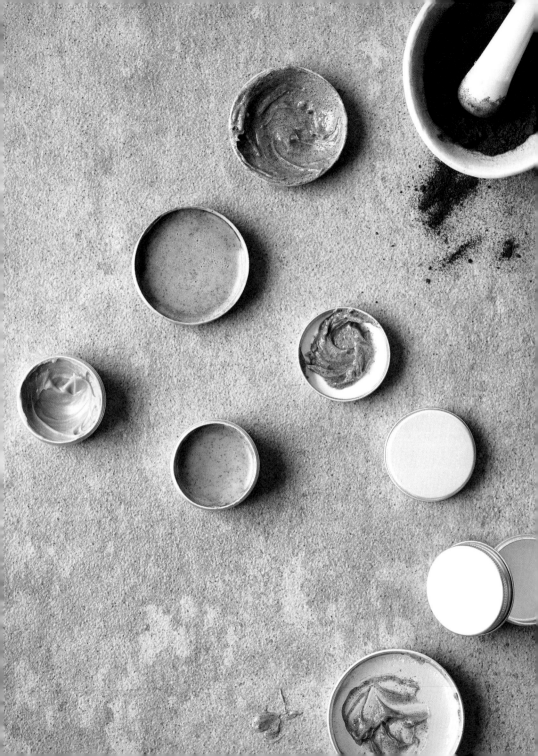

Rose lip balm

I love having coloured lips. It really does make a massive difference to your look and your mood. However, I find it really hard to get my lipstick to stay on and always have really dry lips if I wear it all day. This gloss means I can wear a shade of colour and apply as often as I want without drying out my lips. You can make this in whatever colour you like and they make a lovely little gift. Change the rose to a different smell by just switching the essential oil.

MAKES 125ML

- 4 tablespoons coconut oil
- 2 tablespoons shea butter
- 2 tablespoons beeswax
- 1 teaspoon rose powder or coloured mica powder
- 3–4 drops of rose essential oil

small tin or airtight container with a lid

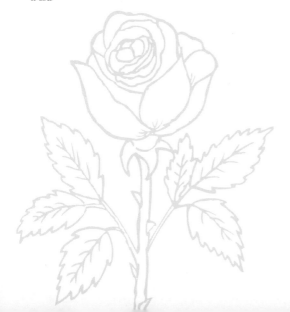

Put the coconut oil, shea butter and beeswax in a double boiler and heat over a low heat, stirring until fully melted. If you don't have a double boiler, then use a heatproof bowl set over a pan of barely simmering water instead (making sure the bottom of the bowl doesn't touch the water underneath).

Remove from the heat and stir in the rose powder or coloured mica powder. Now stir in the rose essential oil. Transfer the mix to a small tin or airtight container, then smooth the top and leave to cool. Once cool, cover and store in a cool, dark place for up to a year.

To use, rub a little of the lip balm over your lips as required.

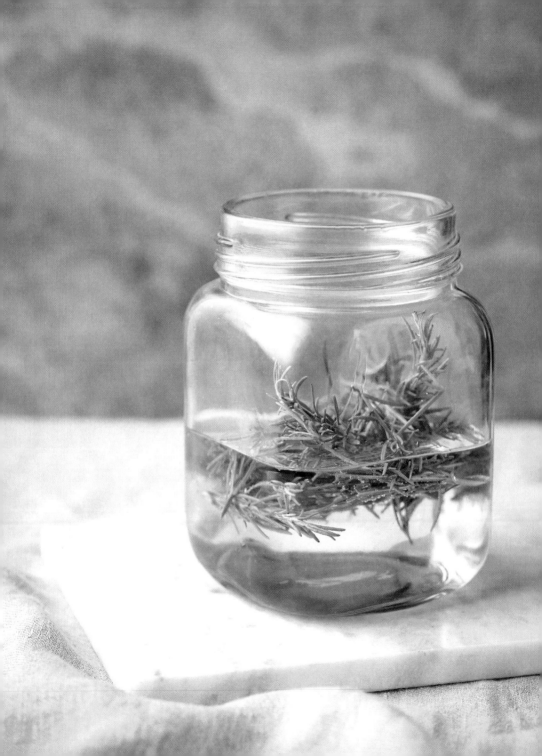

Rosemary face primer

Primer is not really something I use, but I know many people swear by it to help to hold their make-up in place. This recipe was shared with me by a lady called Layla, who attended one of my workshops. It's a beautiful recipe and my friends who tested it said it works a treat and smells delightful, too.

For the rosemary water

MAKES 150ML

6 large sprigs of rosemary
200ml filtered water, to cover

sterilised small jar

Place the rosemary sprigs in a small saucepan and cover with the filtered water. Bring gently to the boil, then simmer for 5 minutes. Remove from the heat and leave to cool, then strain into a sterilised small jar and cover with the lid. Store in a cool, dark place for up to a year. Once opened, store in the fridge and use within a few months.

For the face primer

MAKES 100ML

120ml Rosemary Water (see
 above)
1 teaspoon bicarbonate of soda
3 tablespoons rose water
1 tablespoon witch hazel

sterilised airtight container or jar

Pour the rosemary water into a saucepan and heat gently until warm, then slowly stir in the bicarbonate of soda. Remove from the heat, add the remaining ingredients and stir to combine. Pour into a sterilised airtight container or jar and cover. Store in a cool, dark place for up to 3 months. Shake before use.

To use, pour a teaspoonful of the primer onto a cotton pad and wipe over your face prior to applying your foundation.

Foundation

As a teenager I used to clog my pores with layers and layers of foundation. This recipe won't give you the coverage you are used to with big brand foundation but your skin will thank you.

MAKES ABOUT 50ML

1 teaspoon shea butter

2 teaspoons argan oil or jojoba oil

½ teaspoon emulsifying wax

1 tablespoon aloe vera gel

1 teaspoon witch hazel

½–1 teaspoon cacao powder

½ teaspoon mica powder in your preferred colour (optional)

Melt the shea butter, argan oil and emulsifying wax in a double boiler or a heatproof bowl set over a saucepan of simmering water until completely melted. Add the aloe vera gel and witch hazel and whisk until completely incorporated. Take off the heat. Add the cacao powder (and mica, if using) a little at a time until you reach the colour you desire. Once cool, test the colour and coverage on your cheek. Spoon the mixture into a small airtight container and use as needed. Store for up to a month.

Blusher

My brothers have always teased me about how much blusher I wear. I love it. There is no particular reason, it is just the one thing I always wear and that will never change. If you are fair skinned, reduce the amount of cacao powder.

MAKES ENOUGH FOR 1 MONTH

1 tablespoon arrowroot powder

1 teaspoon raw cacao powder

1 teaspoon coloured mica powder or Floral Powder (see page 42) of your choice, or enough to achieve your desired shade

Mix the arrowroot and cacao powders together thoroughly in a small bowl. Gradually blend in the mica powder or floral powder of your choice until you achieve your desired shade of blusher. Store in an airtight container in a cool, dry place for up to a month.

Apply in the same way as you would regular blusher.

small airtight container

Face powder

For those who are comfortable with no foundation but like a tiny bit of coverage from time to time, or indeed have a spot of shiny skin, this powder is perfect applied straight over your moisturiser or mixed into your foundation. You can adjust the cacao powder to suit your skin tone. Play around with quantities until you get the best shade for your skin. Each option below makes enough for approximately 1–2 months. This can be used as an all over body bronzer too.

MAKES ENOUGH FOR
1–2 MONTHS
for pale skin

4 tablespoons arrowroot powder
½ teaspoon raw cacao powder
2–3 drops of vitamin E oil or
  wheatgerm oil

for tan skin

6 tablespoons arrowroot powder
3 tablespoons raw cacao powder
2–3 drops of vitamin E oil or
  wheatgerm oil

for dark skin

4 tablespoons arrowroot powder
5 tablespoons raw cacao powder
2–3 drops of vitamin E oil or
  wheatgerm oil

airtight container or jar

Place all the ingredients for your skin type into a coffee or spice grinder and blitz to a fine powder, making sure everything is thoroughly mixed. Transfer to an airtight container or jar and close the lid. Store in a cool, dry place for up to 3 months.

To use, either apply a little (as needed) directly over your moisturiser or mix into your foundation before applying as needed.

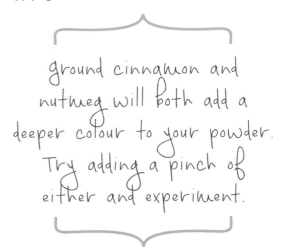

ground cinnamon and nutmeg will both add a deeper colour to your powder. Try adding a pinch of either and experiment.

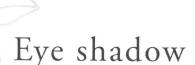

Eye shadow

This recipe is the same as the blusher so it's really simple. You can omit the cacao powder if you want a really vibrant eye shadow. Mica powders come in literally every colour of the rainbow. For more shine, use less arrowroot and more mica.

MAKES ENOUGH
FOR 1 MONTH

1 tablespoon arrowroot powder

½ teaspoon raw cacao powder

1 teaspoon coloured mica powder (whichever colour you like) or Floral Powder (see page 42) of your choice, or enough to achieve your desired shade

small airtight container

Mix the arrowroot and cacao powders together thoroughly in a small bowl. Gradually blend in the mica powder or floral powder of your choice until you achieve your desired shade of eye shadow. Store in an airtight container in a cool, dry place for up to a month.

Apply in the same way as you would with regular eye shadow.

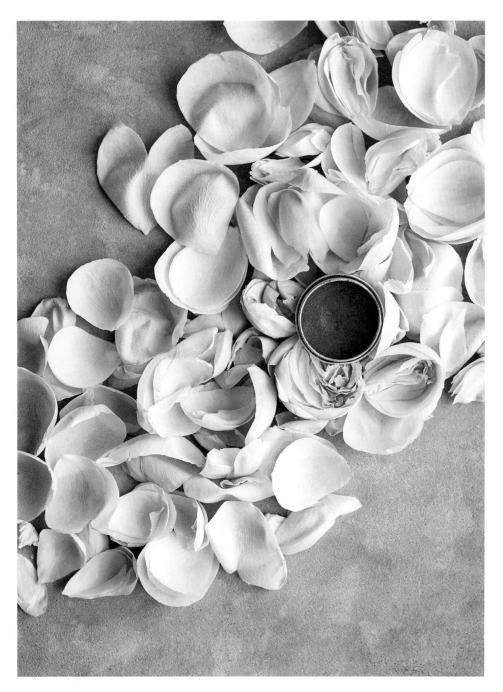

You can easily dry out your own flowers by picking the petals and laying them outside on a cloth, out of direct sunlight, until dry.

Floral powders

For fragrance in talc or colouring in make-up, these powders add a hit of colour and smell delightful! Play around with the colours and flower choice and don't be afraid to give something not listed here a go. Use these petal powders in place of mica powders in eye shadows (see page 40) and blushers (see page 38).

DRIED FLOWER PETALS
SUCH AS:
calendula (for colour)
cornflowers (for colour)
dahlias (for colour)
hibiscus (for colour)
jasmine (for fragrance)
lavender (for fragrance and colour)
marigolds (for colour)
roses (for fragrance and colour)
yarrow (for fragrance and colour)

airtight container

Make sure your chosen petals are crispy dry.

Once they are ready, place the dried petals in small batches into a spice grinder and blitz until you get a fine powder. Store in airtight containers in a cool, dry place for up to a year. Use as required.

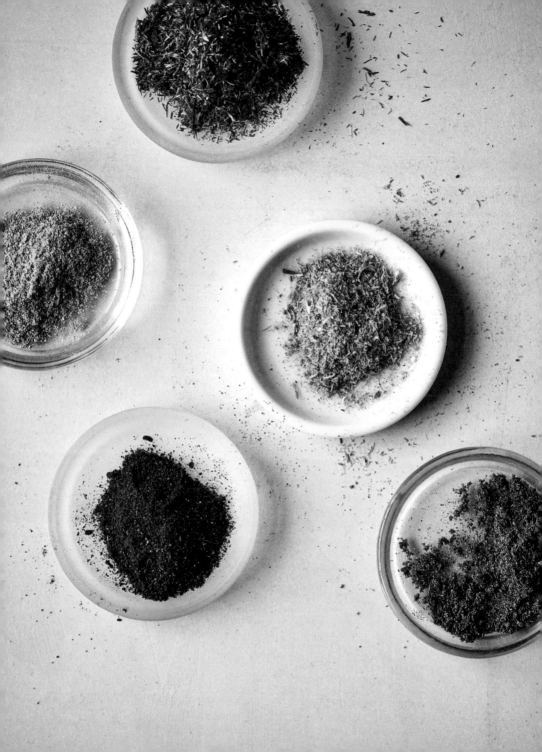

Chapter Three
body

Chocolate orange body butter

This dreamy body butter is wonderful to smell on your skin. The cacao butter is great for elasticity, the shea is good for scars and blemishes, the coconut oil is good for moisture, and the cacao powder (apart from the smell) is the perfect antioxidant addition. The orange oil is uplifting and is said to help with anxiety and depression as well as being anti-ageing.

MAKES 200ML

4 tablespoons cacao butter
2 tablespoons shea butter
2 tablespoons coconut oil
2 teaspoons raw cacao powder
20 drops of orange essential oil

sterilised jar or airtight container

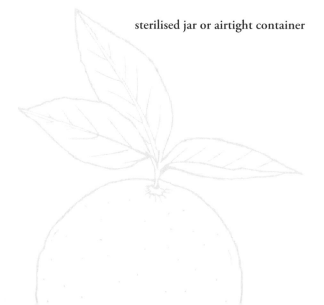

Melt the cacao and shea butters in a double boiler over a low heat. If you don't have a double boiler, use a heatproof bowl set over a pan of barely simmering water instead (making sure the bottom of the bowl doesn't touch the water underneath). Add the coconut oil and leave until melted, then stir to combine. Remove from the heat, add the remaining ingredients and stir to mix. Leave to cool.

Once the mix is cool and solid, transfer it to the bowl of a stand mixer and whip for 8 minutes, or until light and fluffy.

Transfer the whipped butter to a sterilised jar or airtight container. Store in a cool, dark place for up to 3 months. In colder climates, it may solidify, but will warm up enough to melt when it's applied to your skin. In warmer environments, it will become less fluffy over time, but still works a treat.

To use, lightly rub the body butter over your skin, as required.

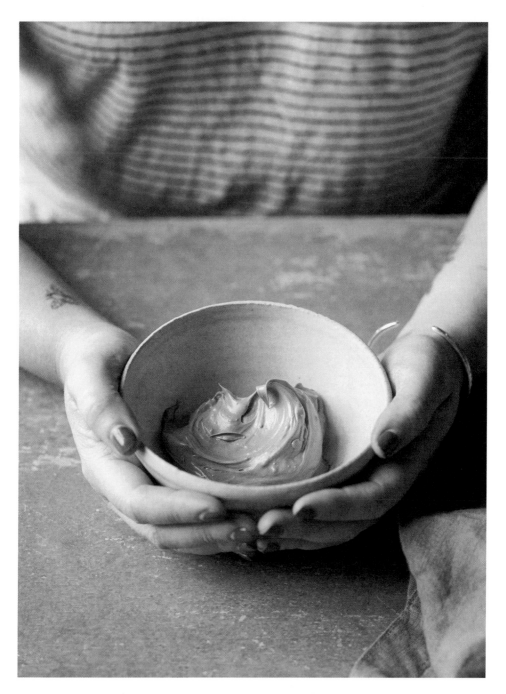

Med-ready body scrub

Even if you're just dreaming of a Mediterranean holiday, you can still have shiny Med-ready skin and feel like you're in the fifth village of Cinque Terre in Italy, drinking a Negroni. Sage and lemon will bring the aroma of all the wonderful summery Sicilian dreams to you in this scrub.

MAKES 120G

1 teaspoon coconut oil

2 teaspoons extra virgin olive oil

120g coarse sea salt

AND

10 drops of mint essential oil

3 drops of lemon essential oil

3 drops of orange essential oil

3 drops of sage essential oil

OR

no essential oils and

zest of 1 lemon

zest of 1 orange

2 sprigs of sage, ripped into small pieces

2 sprigs of mint, ripped into small pieces

sterilised jar with a lid

Melt the coconut and olive oils together in a double boiler over a low heat. If you don't have a double boiler, use a heatproof bowl set over a pan of barely simmering water instead (making sure the bottom of the bowl doesn't touch the water underneath). Remove from the heat.

Place the salt in a bowl with either your essential oils or the zest and herbs. Add the blended oil, a little at a time, stirring slowly until combined. You may not need to use all the oil – it depends on the consistency you're after. Don't overmix or it will become runny.

Transfer the scrub mix to a sterilised jar, close the lid and store the jar in the shower. This body scrub will keep for 2–3 months.

To use, spread the body scrub over wet skin, massaging liberally, then rinse with warm water.

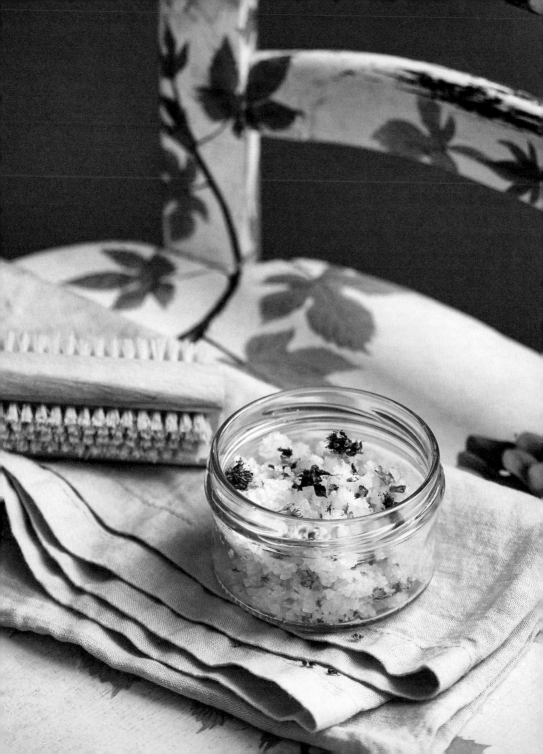

Apricot & vanilla body custard

Honestly, if you put this next to a bowl of custard, you wouldn't know the difference. I love this recipe. Apricot kernel oil is so rich in essential fatty acids and is best for dry skin. It is also super high in vitamin A.

MAKES 250G

120ml apricot kernel oil

4 tablespoons shea butter

4 tablespoons coconut oil, melted

1 vanilla pod, split lengthways and seeds scraped out

sterilised jar

Place everything in a blender or use a hand-held blender in a bowl and blitz for a minute or so until emulsified.

Pour into a sterilised jar, close the lid and leave to set in the fridge. This will keep in the fridge for up to 3 months.

To use, lightly rub the body custard over your skin, as required.

Natural deodorant

This may or may not work for you. Sadly, I suffer from smelly underarms so I tend to buy natural deodorant instead of making my own, but some of my friends have had real success with this and similar recipes. Lucky you who smell like roses… Give it a try. Every person is different.

MAKES 100G

50g bicarbonate of soda

50g arrowroot powder

10 drops of essential oil of your choice (try tea tree, lavender or rosemary)

about 4 tablespoons coconut oil

airtight container

In a small bowl, mix together the bicarbonate of soda, arrowroot and essential oil to make a smooth paste. Begin to incorporate the coconut oil, a little at a time, stirring continuously until you have a paste thick enough to spread on your skin. Transfer the mix to an airtight container to stop it from drying out. Store in a cool, dry place for up to six months. Use as required by wiping a little of the mix onto your clean armpits using your fingers.

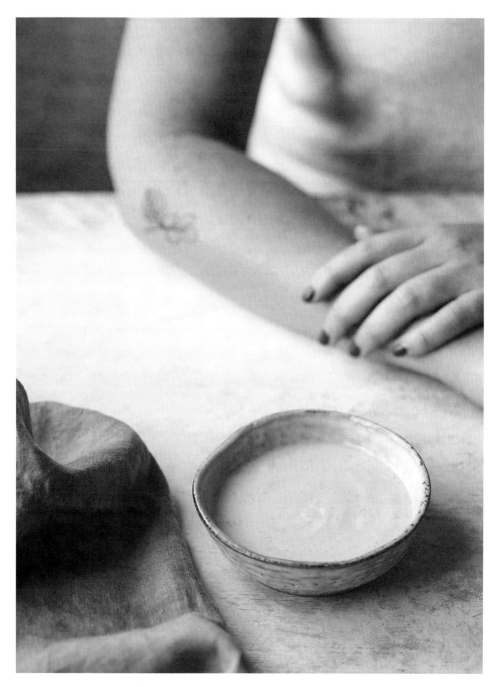

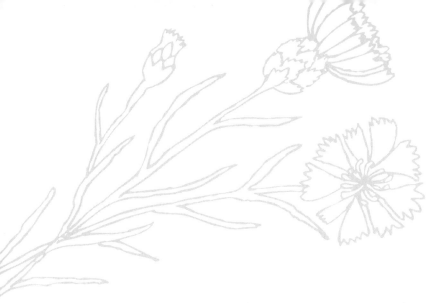

Flower not-talcum powder

Talc reminds me of my great grandma, Lil, the talc queen. Little did she know quite how toxic her after-bath powdering really was. It is not good for you at all to breathe in and has been linked to all kinds of nasty diseases and environmental concerns. This is my homemade, natural alternative. Orris root powder is a fixative, so it helps to keep the scent in the powder for longer. It's often used in potpourri for this reason, but you don't have to use it here.

MAKES 320G

250g arrowroot powder (you can use cornflour instead, but it's less silky)

3–4 tablespoons Floral Powder of your choice (see page 42)

1 tablespoon orris root powder

small jar or airtight container

Mix everything together in a bowl, then transfer to a small jar or airtight container and cover. Store in a cool, dry place for up to a year.

After you have showered or bathed and are towel-dry, use by applying it with a powder brush, as required.

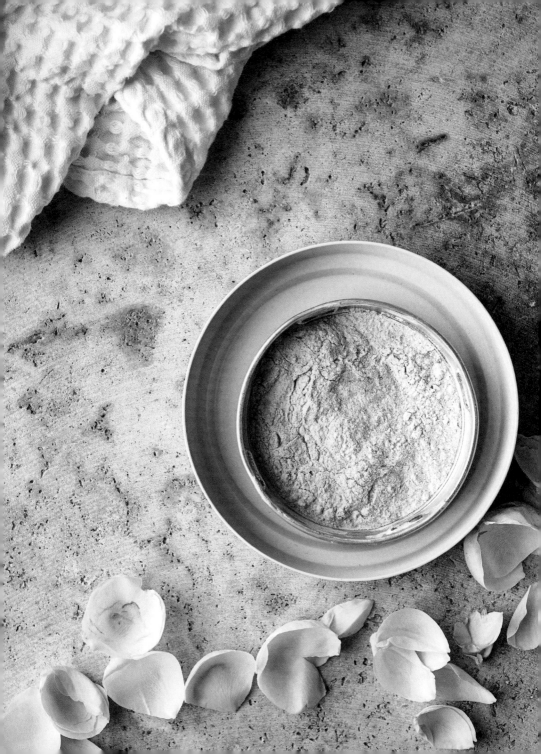

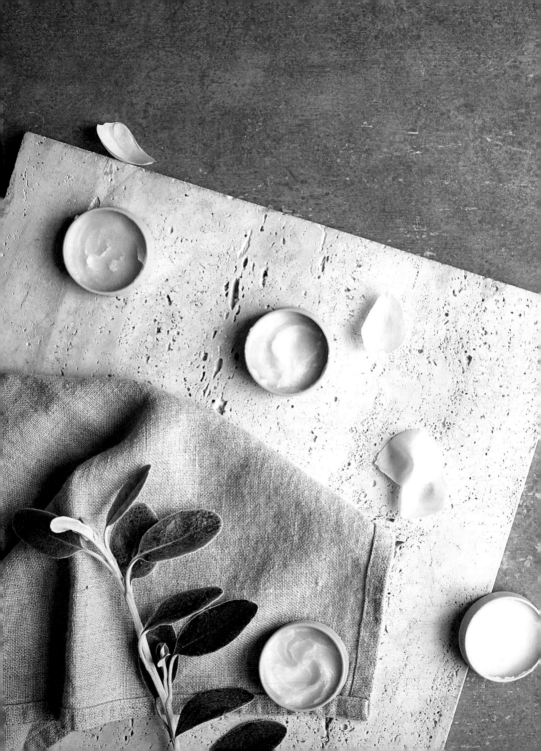

Perfume pots

Solid perfumes are an easy way to make your own fragrances that actually last on your skin. This is the easiest recipe and will allow you to play around with essential oils until you find the combination you love. Go ahead and be an alchemist.

MAKES 30ML

1 tablespoon beeswax

1 tablespoon coconut oil

a few drops of natural food colouring or a sprinkle of mica powder (optional, if you want to colour your perfume)

20–30 drops of essential oils in any combination you like

TRY:

Orange – to uplift and energise

Lavender – to calm and relieve stress

Rose – to ease emotional blockages and stress

Frankincense – to uplift and ground

Ginger – to uplift and energise

Jasmine – for peace and tranquility

small lip gloss container or jar

Melt the beeswax and coconut oil in a double boiler over a low heat. If you don't have a double boiler, use a heatproof bowl set over a pan of barely simmering water instead (making sure the bottom of the bowl doesn't touch the water underneath). Remove from the heat and slowly add the food colouring or mica powder, if using, and the essential oils, stirring as you go.

Pour into a small lip gloss container or jar, cover and leave to set, then voilà – perfume, handbag ready. Store in a cool, dry place for up to a year.

To use, simply dab a little of the perfume behind your ears, on your temples or wherever you normally apply perfume.

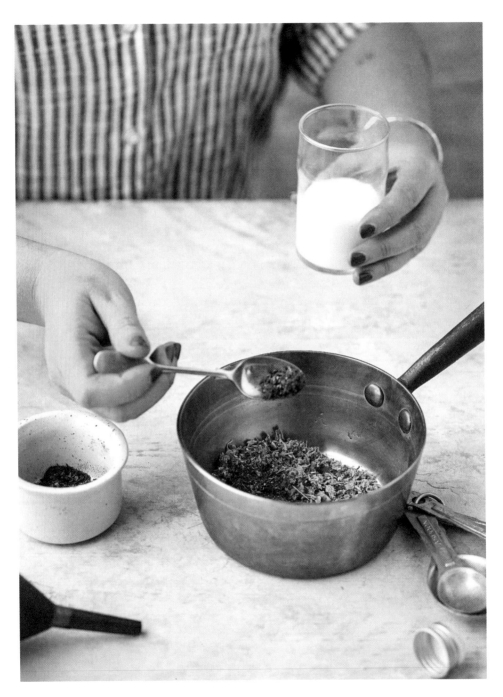

Milk, marshmallow and violet after-sun

Marshmallow leaf and violets are emollients, which means they are soothing on sore and burnt skin. The addition of milk and aloe, two other powerful emollients, makes for a chemical-free solution to sunburn. Much easier and better for us to not get burnt in the first place, though.

MAKES 75ML

50ml whole milk

**1 teaspoon dried violets or
    2 teaspoons fresh**

**1 teaspoon dried marshmallow
    leaf**

1 tablespoon aloe vera oil

sterilised small spray bottle

Place the milk, violets and marshmallow leaf in a small saucepan and bring gently to the boil. Remove from the heat, then stir in the aloe oil until combined. Cover and leave to cool.

Strain into a sterilised small spray bottle and put in the fridge. This spray will keep in the fridge for up to a week, so make it in small batches as needed.

To use, lightly spray the after-sun over sunburnt skin, as required.

Always wear sunscreen. This recipe will soothe a mild sunburn, but for anything more serious, seek medical attention.

Chapter Four
hair

Shampoo

Coconut is the perfect moisturiser and will leave your hair silky smooth, while the orange essential oil makes you smell good enough to eat. Who doesn't want that?

MAKES ABOUT 120ML
(enough for about 4 washes, depending on the length of your hair)

60ml coconut milk, canned or homemade

60ml liquid castile soap

20 drops of orange essential oil (optional)

½ teaspoon olive oil or nut oil (optional, for dry hair)

recycled shampoo bottle or an airtight container or screw-top jar

Combine all the ingredients in a recycled shampoo bottle or an airtight container or screw-top jar. Shake well to mix. Store in your shower for up to a month. Just remember to shake well before every use, and use as required.

If you suffer from dandruff,
try swapping the orange oil for tea tree
or eucalyptus oil.

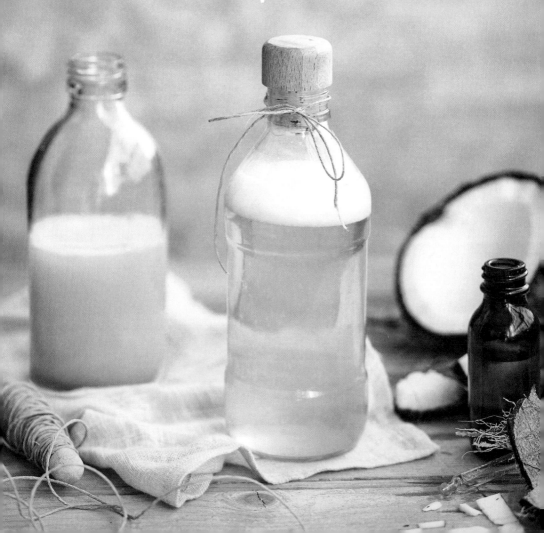

Coconut conditioner

This gorgeous conditioner will leave your hair extra smooth. First use pure coconut oil to moisturise and condition, then follow through with the 50:50 mixture of apple cider vinegar and water as a rinse, to really clean your hair and help with scalp problems, such as dandruff. The acid removes any excess oil from your hair and increases its shine. Try using it once a week or so.

MAKES 1 APPLICATION

1–2 teaspoons coconut oil, in a
   liquid state
60ml raw apple cider vinegar
60ml water
10 drops of essential oil of
   your choice
TRY:
Sage – for normal hair
Tea tree – for oily hair
Lavender – for dandruff

airtight container or screw-top jar

Make sure the coconut oil is liquid – place it in a warm place to melt if need be.

Put the vinegar, water and essential oil in an airtight container or screw-top jar. Shake well to mix. You can make a larger quantity of this vinegar rinse and keep it in your shower for up to a month, if you like – just remember to shake well before every use.

After you have washed your hair, start by rubbing the coconut oil into the ends of your hair and then leave for a few minutes. Rinse thoroughly in warm water. Pour the vinegar mix through your hair and rinse thoroughly.

Arrowroot powder rubbed into the roots of your hair works well for a quick refresh. If you have light hair, use it on its own. For dark hair, add a little raw cacao before use.

Dry shampoo

I am the queen of dry shampoo. I have been known (OK, I have not *been* known, I *am* known) for being a once-a-week washer of my hair. Yet I have always had a real problem using dry shampoo because they come in an aerosol can. It's been a recent discovery that I can now make my own without a can. It's like winning the lottery.

Kaolin clay is a white cosmetic clay that is known for its absorbency and removal of dirt and oil, which means it is also great for acne-prone skin. Kaolin clay is readily available online.

MAKES ENOUGH FOR 2–5 APPLICATIONS (depending on the thickness of your hair

1 teaspoon kaolin clay

1 teaspoon arrowroot powder

(if you have dark hair, add ½–1 teaspoon ground cinnamon or ½–1 teaspoon raw cacao powder)

small jar with a lid

Put everything through a sieve into a small jar. Add cinnamon or cacao powder as needed, depending on the darkness of your hair. Poke holes in the lid for easy application. Shake the mix into your roots as needed and brush through.

Store in a cool, dry place for up to 6 months.

Salty macadamia hair spritz

You might not expect this, but salt is actually an incredible hydrator. It is also wonderful for that just-went-for-a-quick-surf-before-work look. The macadamia oil helps to keep the hair extra nourished.

MAKES 280ML

250ml boiled water, cooled to warm
1 tablespoon good-quality salt
1 tablespoon macadamia oil

recycled spray bottle

Pour the warm water into a jug and stir in the salt until completely dissolved, then stir in the macadamia oil. Pour into a recycled spray bottle, then shake before each use. Store in a cool, dark place and use within 3 months.

To use, spritz onto wet or dry hair, keeping your eyes closed, as often as needed.

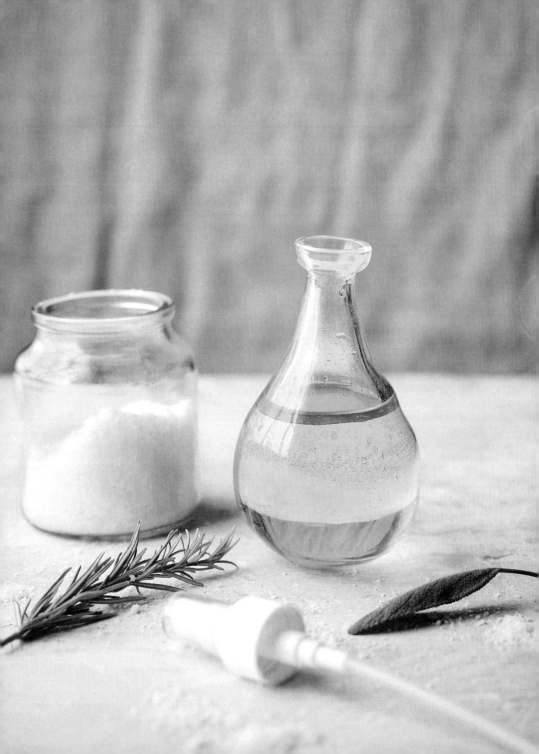

Hair masks three ways

My hair is extremely thick and very dry. It's dry because my hair is coloured (not very natural, I know, but nobody is perfect). I love to dye my hair and I change it far too often. Because of this I need a hair mask from time to time. Here are a few different masks for every kind of hair.

To treat dry hair

Raw honey is one of the most nourishing ingredients that exists in the natural world so is perfect to add moisture and shine.

MAKES 1 APPLICATION

5 tablespoons raw honey
60ml water

Mix the honey and water together in a small bowl. Rub the mix through your damp hair. Leave for 10 minutes, then rinse with warm water and wash as normal.

To treat oily hair

Kaolin clay is an absorbent so will draw oil from the roots of your hair.

MAKES 1 APPLICATION

150ml green tea, brewed, strained and cooled to warm
5 tablespoons kaolin clay

Make a paste by combining the green tea and kaolin clay in a small bowl. Rub the mix into the scalp on wet hair. Leave for 10 minutes, then rinse with warm water and wash as normal.

To give hair shine

Eggs are full of protein and hair packed with protein means shiny locks.

MAKES 1 APPLICATION

2 egg yolks
120ml apple cider vinegar

Whisk the egg yolks in a small bowl, then work them through clean but wet hair using a comb. Rinse with lukewarm water (not hot water, otherwise your hair will end up with scrambled eggs in it), then pour over the vinegar and rinse again.

Chapter Five

hands

Honey hands

This is so moisturising. It makes the most wonderful overnight treatment. Rub a generous amount onto your hands before bed and put on some disposable gloves to lock in the moisture. If using as hand cream it feels a little sticky at first but soon dissipates. This is also great used on shabby cuticles.

MAKES 140ML
(for an overnight treatment)

2 tablespoons shea butter
1 tablespoon coconut oil
2 tablespoons raw honey
2 tablespoons argan oil
20 drops of rose or rosehip
   essential oil

sterilised jar or airtight container

Melt the shea butter and coconut oil in a double boiler over a low heat. If you don't have a double boiler, use a heatproof bowl set over a pan of barely simmering water instead (making sure the bottom of the bowl doesn't touch the water underneath).

Stir in the honey, then remove from the heat and stir in the argan oil and the essential oil. Leave to cool.

Once the mix is cool, transfer it to the bowl of a stand mixer and whip for 4–6 minutes, or until light and fluffy. You can use a hand-held mixer too.

Transfer the whipped mix to a sterilised jar or airtight container and cover. Store in a cool, dark place for up to 3 months.

To use, lightly rub the creamy mix over your cuticles and hands, as often as required.

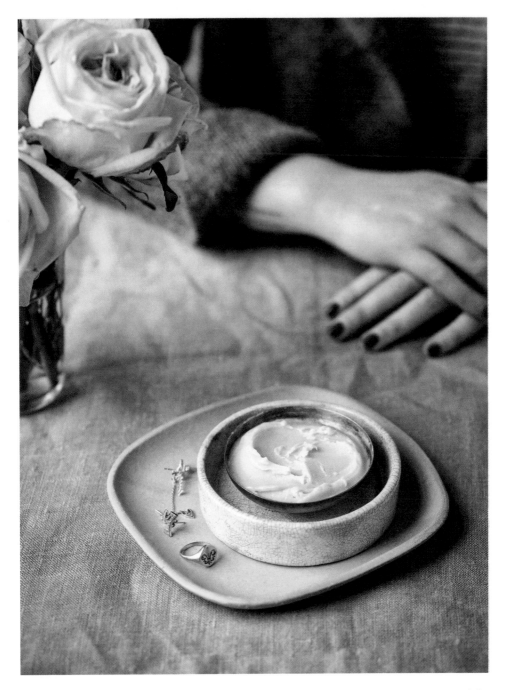

Herby hand sanitiser

Let it be known that I am absolutely anti-antibacterial hand sanitisers. Thay have gone from being used in emergency rooms to being in every minor interaction. This causes the same problem as using antibiotics at the first sign of any illness – it doesn't actually help our bodies to deal with illness or infection, and we end up with weaker immune systems. 'Antibacterial' also means anti all types of bacteria, so good bacteria will be killed too. This recipe is to clean, not to kill.

MAKES 120ML

100ml aloe vera gel

20ml nut oil

10 drops thyme essential oil

10 drops lavender essential oil

10 drops eucalyptus essential oil

5 drops tea tree essential oil

sterilised pump bottle

In a bowl, whisk together the aloe and nut oil until emulsification begins. Add the essential oils and whisk again until well combined.

Spoon into a sterilised pump bottle or your chosen bottle. Keep sealed, as it will evaporate if left open.

Apply to your hands as needed and rub into the skin. This will keep for up to 6 months.

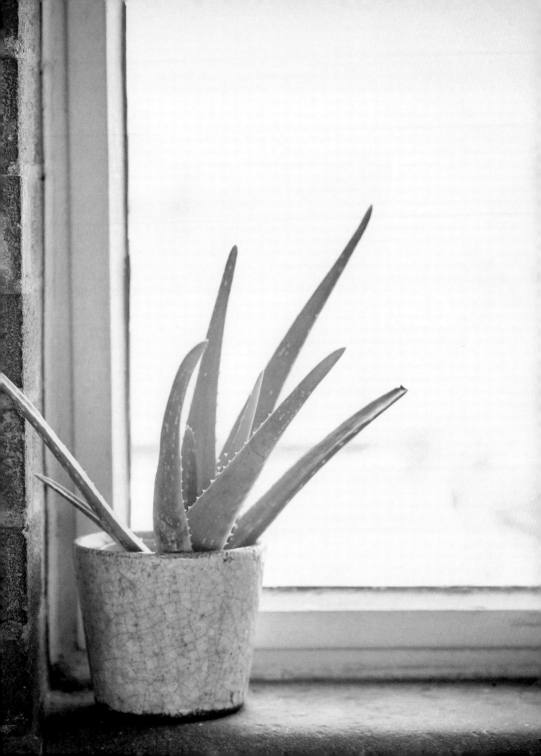

Resources

Below are just some of the fantastic suppliers you can source your ingredients and equipment from.

WORLDWIDE DELIVERY

New Directions

For cosmetic bases, essential oils, castile soap, bottles and jars, packaging and dried ingredients
www.newdirections.com.au

Amazon

For cosmetic bases, essential oils, carrier oils, castile soap, bottles and jars, packaging and dried ingredients
www.amazon.co.uk or
www.amazon.com

Bulk Apothecary

For cosmetic bases, essential oils, castile soap, bottles and jars, packaging and dried ingredients
www.bulkapothecary.com

Baldwins

For cosmetic bases, essential oils, castle soap, bottles and jars, packaging and dried ingredients
www.baldwins.co.uk

Wholesale Mineral Makeup

For mica and make up ingredients, with worlwide delivery
www.wholesalemineralmakeup.com.au

Speciality Bottle

Bottles and cosmetic equipment
www.specialtybottle.com

Organic alcohol

Alcohol for tinctures and tonics
www.organicalcohol.com

UK

Neal's Yard
 For dried herbs, essential oils and
 carrier oils
 www.nealsyardremedies.com
Pestle Herbs
 For fried Herbs and apothecary bottles
 www.pestleherbs.co.uk

AUSTRALIA

Austral Herbs
 For dried herbs and flowers
 www.australherbs.com.au
Essentially Australia
 For essential oils
 www. essentiallyaustralia.com.au

USA & CANADA

Mountain Rose Herbs
 For dried herbs and flowers
 www.mountainroseherbs.com

Index

Index continued

Acknowledgements

Firstly to my family. My mum and dad have always supported me and I love that they sit in what my dad calls his 'proud chair' because of the path I am on. All I have ever wanted was to make them and my brothers proud. So to you my small family and the rest of my big extended family, especially its oh so wonderful leader my nan (and great grandmother Lil). To all of you, Sarah, Nigel, Paul, Mark, Kylie, Skye, Angie, Bec, Harry, Nicole,Yasmin, Sam, Teryn, Ashleigh, Caitlyn, Liam, Brad and Taylah and then the rest of our little family Emma, Koen and my godsons Charlie and Rory. You are all everything to me. As are you Damien, my love. Thank you for putting up with our home looking like a constant laboratory and test kitchen. To my friends who have supported me for decades.

To Kyle. I have no words to express how grateful I am to you. To our new Octopus family, here is to a long journey making beautiful and meaningful books together. To my team. The A team. Tara, the most incredible Editor a girl could ask for. Your patience, generosity and passion for these next books made them what they are. Nassima. Thank you for making my recipes and creations come to life. I only hope we work on many a more things together. Rachel. No words can thank you enough for being the most incredible partner in crime styling these books and seeing inside my messy brain. You are so immensely talented and I am so grateful. Agathe, Laura and the rest of the team. High fives all round! To all of the people in my work world who have taught me so very much over the years. Thank you. There is no way I would be where I am without you teaching me everything I know. Last but not at all least, to all of you who bought this book.
    Massive gratitude from the bottom of my heart.

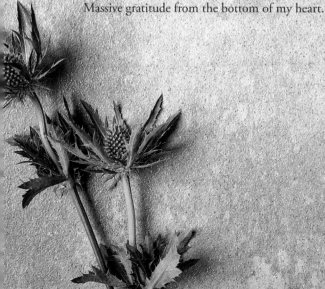